Made in the USA
Coppell, TX
21 July 2022

80251016R00061